Dress Thin!
330 Tips

Fashion is architecture; it is a matter of proportion.

Coco Chanel

This is an eye-opening read! With all the emphasis on body image, why not just follow some simple fashion tricks that work? I even use this book in my training seminars for professional women.

Mary Jo Carlson
Hilton Head, South Carolina

Ladies — read this book and discover how to look thin instantly. You need this book right now. Don't we all?

Cynthia Geletka
Potomac, Maryland

Forget the South Beach Diet, forget Atkins — and buy *Dress Thin!* This book really works.

Linda Miller
Westport, Connecticut

I love the user-friendly format of this book. These two authors have become my favorite fashion police. In fact, I've bought *Dress Thin!* for just about every woman I know.

Nancy Ponturo
Redding, Connecticut

If the reader gets even one good tip from this book — it's worth the price. *Dress Thin!* encouraged me to accept myself for the way I am. It also gave me the courage to really improve and update my wardrobe.

Chrissy Rickard
Menard, Texas

Dress Thin!
330 Tips

*How to Use Clothing and Accessories
to Flatter Your Figure*

Jeanne M. Dallman
and
Rose Mary Dallman

BRAINSTORM BOOKS
P.O. Box 1005
Thousand Oaks, CA 91358-1005

Published by:
BRAINSTORM BOOKS
P.O. Box 1005
Thousand Oaks, CA 91358-0005

Publisher's Cataloging-in-Publication
(Provided by Quality Books, Inc.)
Dallman, Jeanne M.
 Dress thin! : 330 tips : how to use clothing and accessories to flatter your figure / [Jeanne M. Dallman, Rose Mary Dallman]. — 2nd ed.
 p. cm.
 ISBN: 0-9705757-5-0

 1. Clothing and dress. 2. Fashion. 3. Beauty, Personal.
I. Dallman, Rose Mary. II. Title.
TT507.D352001 646'.3
 QBI00-911

Dress Thin! is available at a special discount when purchased in bulk for Premiums, Sales Promotions and so on. Special Editions or book excerpts can also be arranged. Contact the publisher.

Book Production: Penelope C. Paine
Editing: Gail Kearns
Cover Design: Knockout Design
Book Layout and Typography: Cirrus Design

Manufactured in the United States of America

Dedicated to you, the Reader,
because you deserve to look and feel
your very best right now!

About the Authors

Jeanne M. Dallman is a writer of both non-fiction and fiction, and is a public speaker. She has a Master of Fine Arts degree from UCLA and is an Adjunct Professor of English at Western Connecticut State University.

Rose Mary Dallman, her mother, is a writer of non-fiction. She is a Journalism graduate from Marquette University and has advertising agency experience.

Many thanks particularly to Penelope Paine for her steady guidance, as well as to Gail Kearns, Peri Poloni and Christine Nolt for their excellent contributions to this book.

Introduction

Let's all be honest about something.

Almost every one of us wants to be thin.

Or at least we want to look our very best— regardless of our size.

Well, we can!

Right now!

Immediately.

Simply follow the fashion secrets described in this book and you, too, will begin to look slimmer instantly.

This is not an exaggeration. Fashion designers have known about these design principles and camouflage strategies for decades.

Now it is simply your turn to use them!

It is all about carefully guiding the viewer's eye with the right color, cut and fabric of clothing.

It is also a matter of wearing the right accessory in order to distract and control the unsuspecting eye.

Very simply, it is a matter of optical illusion!

For example, wearing a vertical line in an outfit, such as in a long row of buttons, will make a woman look taller and therefore slimmer.

And, conversely, wearing a two-piece, two-color outfit that meets at the waist will make a woman look shorter and therefore heavier.

There is nothing magical about it.

And yet, maybe there is . . .

Because now you don't have to actually lose those extra pounds in order to look great right away.

You can flatter your figure today!

Just read on and try these simple dressing tips. Some of them will describe common mistakes many women make, and others will address figure flaws that typically need a bit of disguising. Still others will tell you how to emphasize your best assets!

But, whatever the tip, each one is simple and easy to use.

Finally, when you do decide to trust and experiment with these tricks of the trade, you will begin to notice one very important thing.

You are becoming more self-confident . . .

And everyone knows that what really makes a person attractive is a quiet self-confidence.

So do it for yourself.

Don't do it in order to look like someone else or because you think you need to look model-thin.

Do it because you deserve to look your very best right now.

Our Motto:

Look great.
Feel great.
Do great.
Be great.

All the Best,

Jeanne M. Dallman
and
Rose Mary Dallman

It is possible to have lots of clothes and not an ounce of style. It is also possible to have very few clothes and lots of style.

Hara Estroff Marano

1

Vertical lines and patterns in an outfit will always hide unwanted pounds! That is rule number one.

2

Wear baggy clothes on the top or on bottom — but never on both.

3

Clothes should always fit loose and easy at your trouble spots! It is impossible to overstate this rule: Do not wear clothes that are too tight!

4

A long, tailored vest will hide a multitude of problems. Just don't wear it too baggy or too tight.

5

Do not embellish problem areas! Never wear a fancy necklace near a large bust, or a wide belt near a plump tummy.

6

Choose pants tapered in at the bottom. Pants full around the ankles will always shorten and widen a body.

7

Avoid wearing horizontal stripes at all costs! This is a common mistake. Only the very narrowest of stripes that run sideways should be considered.

8

Clothes in soft fabrics that drape well, just skimming the body, are the most flattering. Fabrics can really make all the difference!

It is never too late, in fiction or in life, to revise.
Nancy Thayer

9

To minimize a large bust, avoid breast pockets and double-breasted jackets.

10

When a woman's neck looks long, she appears taller and thinner! Achieve this look by keeping the area around your neck fairly bare and unadorned. Short hair helps also.

11

Heavy legs are best hidden under simple, wide-leg pants — but not too wide. Avoid bulky pockets, pleats and other ornamentation.

12

Always bend way over — and sit down — in any new garment before buying it. Clothes should not ride up in the back or pull tightly across the shoulders, chest or hips.

13

Please don't even think about wearing a fanny pack! Some accessories are better left to the teenagers.

Your clothes speak even before you do.

Jacqueline Murray

14

To hide a large tummy, wear tops that end just below the hipbone.

15

Avoid boxy dresses! Find designs that have a soft tapering in at the waist.

16

Keep collars simple on blouses to de-emphasize an over-large bust.

17

The classic sheath dress with darts almost always slims the figure because it avoids the waist issue.

18

Shoulder pads on coats should not be large. Your coat will already be layered over a blouse, dress or jacket.

Life is a succession of moments. To live each one is to succeed.

Corita Kent

19

The use of strategically placed color panels is a great trick that swimsuit designers use to minimize waist and thigh problems.

20

To balance broad hips, turn your blouse or shirt collar up and out a bit.

21

Need we say it? Women with heavy thighs or calves should bypass miniskirts altogether.

22

If your hips are a problem, wear a vivid color on top.

23

A plump tummy can be nicely hidden under a dropwaist dress. A loose style works best.

I base most of my fashion taste on what doesn't itch!

Gilda Radner

24

Opaque black tights will make heavy legs look thinner.

25

Look for designers that feature separates. This will allow you to buy different size tops and bottoms.

26

Simply improving your posture while sitting or standing can make you look pounds thinner! Comfortable posture bras are also available now. Try one.

27

Stirrup pants are a great addition to your wardrobe. They give a sleek, slimming look. But always hide the stirrups under boots or shoes.

28

A smile is the fastest, most efficient, most inexpensive way to improve your appearance.

There are really only three types of people: those who make things happen, those who watch things happen, and those who say, what happened?

Ann Landers

29

Skirts with a back slit should cover the backs of plump knees.

30

Wearing clothes that have a sense of adventure about them (because of style or color) can actually make you look thinner and younger!

31

The drawstring jacket is figure friendly! It is soft, fluid and long. But remember to keep the silhouette and sleeves on the narrow side.

32

Dots — even small dots — will often add a look of heaviness.

33

Do not carry an overpacked or plump handbag. The person carrying it also looks plump.

Don't wait for your ship to come in. Swim out to it.

Anonymous

34

All but ignore clothing sizes! They aren't standard anyway. Instead, look in a three-way mirror. Turn slowly and really look. Does it fit?

35

Know the widest part of your body — and don't wear tops that end there.

36

Avoid layering clothes too much or the effect is a bulky one. Or layer in soft materials.

37

If you have gained weight, have the courage to weed out the wrong clothes in your closet! If possible, buy a few good quality pieces that really fit and flatter.

38

Never repeat a shape you want to disguise. If your face is round, avoid a round hat. If your face is large and square, avoid a large, square collar or pin.

Who said clothes make a statement? What an understatement that was. Clothes never shut up.

Susan Brownmiller

39

Avoid wearing large earrings and a large necklace at the same time. Keep one of the two small to prevent a busy look.

40

If you decide to wear a subtle print, avoid a white or very light background.

41

A coat dress, with its long, sleek lines and vertical buttons, is always flattering.

42

Fabrics such as velvet, velour and corduroy actually reflect light — and are therefore not recommended. They make a person look larger.

43

Choose a swimsuit that provides a needed distraction. For example, if your hips are a problem, find a suit with a fashion element at the top.

Happiness sneaks through a door you didn't know you left open.

John Barrymore

44

Never let a shoulder bag hang at the widest part of your body! It will widen your silhouette further. Adjust the strap or don't buy it.

45

Avoid heavily patterned, splashy print tops and dresses. Such busyness inevitably adds pounds.

46

Fur is not only controversial — it is usually bulky, which adds girth.

47

Beware of knits however comfortable they may be. Knits tend to cling and are very unforgiving.

48

Talk with experienced salespeople. Wardrobe consultants are often available in shops and department stores. They can be a valuable resource when analyzing your own figure strengths and flaws.

Everybody is the architect of his own fortune.

German Proverb

49

A round face will appear more slim and better proportioned when hair is parted in the middle.

50

Wear coats a bit on the long side. This is important.

51

If you look best in classic, tailored clothes, consider yourself lucky! Simplicity is slimming.

52

Do not wear platform shoes! In fact, avoid all chunky footwear altogether. Simple, low-cut classic pumps help legs look longer.

53

If you are broad shouldered, be careful of shoulder pads. Don't hesitate to remove them from clothing.

It is a funny thing about life: if you refuse to accept anything but the best you very often get it.

William Somerset Maugham

54

Seek out the magical jumper! Not only does it provide a vertical line, it is feminine as well.

55

Find a skilled tailor! Create, alter and update your clothes anew!

56

Beaded, angora sweaters are best left to the small-busted woman.

57

When a trench coat is relaxed — and the fabric, belt and details are softened — all women can look chic.

58

Diagonal lines in an outfit or fabric are also vertical lines — which means they are flattering. In addition, they are attractive and full of energy.

Few women are born beautiful but every woman can aspire to attractiveness.

Hara Estroff Marano

59

If you have a short neck, wear a collarless jacket or coat.

60

Women with heavy legs should always try to match hosiery and footwear to their skirts and dresses.

61

Unless thighs are a problem, straight, slim trouser legs will make you look taller and thinner.

62

If you love to wear a sweatsuit — do so — but be careful of the fabric: it shouldn't be too thin or too thick. And the fit should be just right. You may need to spend some extra money on this item.

63

The shawl collar — whether on a dress, sweater, jacket or coat — lengthens, and therefore slenderizes, one's figure.

Knowing is not enough; we must apply. Willing is not enough; we must do.

Johann Wolfgang von Goethe

64

Keep in mind that a short jacket that stops in the middle of the hip will cut the body in half and widen it.

65

If you have a waist problem, wear pants and skirts that zip on the side or in back. You won't believe the difference!

66

Women with thick calves and ankles should wear long, lean boots.

67

Find the middle ground! Clothes too voluminous will make you look unshapely — but clothes too fitted will highlight your curves.

68

A straight cardigan jacket with a V-neck is wonderfully flattering. Find one with great buttons and wear it over just about any skirt or pants.

We all have possibilities we don't know about. We can do things we don't even dream we can do.

Dale Carnegie

69

A mock, not bulky, turtleneck can help minimize a heavy neck or double chin.

70

Stick to wearing one substantial accessory instead of a group of them. Remember, less is more.

71

Lots of great, new high tech fabrics are available now! For example, the Lycra/stretch Coolmax fabric will stretch practically forever without losing its shape. Also look for a Lycra/nylon blend or a Lycra/cotton blend.

72

Usually select clothes that are slightly fitted.

73

The V-neck pullover sweater can look great on every figure type! Wear it long, of course, but not wide or sloppy.

Simplicity is the ultimate sophistication.

Leonardo da Vinci

74

Avoid frilly tops — especially if your bust is large.

75

Stay away from bulky sweaters altogether. They add width where they shouldn't.

76

Short (not droopy) straps in a swimsuit will help pull you up and tame an ample breast. So will wide straps. Also consider an underwire.

77

A tea-length hemline often flatters a woman's figure. It provides a nice vertical line.

78

Should you wear a belt? Put one on. If it rides up, don't wear it. But, remember, a belt does not help lengthen the figure.

He has good judgment who relies not wholly on his own.

English Proverb

79

Minimize an over-ample bustline by wearing semi-wide pant legs.

80

Be aware of your coat size! It must fit gracefully over tops, sweaters and dresses. A cramped, too small size gives a heavy look.

81

In general, wear dark colors where you want to look smaller — and light colors where your proportions are pleasing.

82

If you are ample on top, do not wear cropped tops or short, tight sweaters.

83

If you are a bit heavy in the mid-section, pants with a simple waistline in front and an elasticized band in the back can be great looking.

We tend to get what we expect.
                                    Norman Vincent Peale

84

A collarless style of jacket always works well on the large-breasted woman.

85

If your waist is a problem, accentuate your shoulders.

86

The underwire bra, with its uplift and support, is an excellent choice for the ample-busted woman.

87

You can find great T-shirts now with small, built-in shoulder pads to help balance your figure. This type of pad won't bunch up or travel.

88

If you are wide-hipped, the boatneck sweater can help balance your proportions.

Good counsel never comes too late.

German Proverb

89

Gloves can make a great distracting statement, especially colorful ones! The longer the better.

90

Be careful of sleeves that are too tight. This rule applies no matter how long the sleeve.

91

Light-colored pantyhose widens the leg. Darker shades are more slimming. Avoid white altogether.

92

If your arms are slender and you want to direct the viewer's eye upward, try pushing up your blouse sleeves.

93

Enhancing your makeup is worth the effort and money — especially for the woman who is a bit heavy. But it is difficult to do well. Take the time to consult a makeup professional.

Never too late to learn.

Scottish Proverb

94

Bodyshapers are available in lingerie departments and will definitely hide unwanted pounds. Because they're made of stretchy Lycra, they are very efficient at trimming waistlines, hips, thighs and derrieres.

95

If your face is plump or wide, wear flat earrings rather than bulky ones.

96

Be very careful with glitter and fancy clothing decorations. Understate, understate. Go for a trim, classic look.

97

When wearing skirts, be aware of your
hemline! A large tummy can make it ride
up in the back. Re-hem the skirt or at least
tuck up the waistband in front.

98

If your derriere is a bit large, avoid partial
belts in the back of a dress, jacket or coat.

*You can be pleased with nothing when you are not
pleased with yourself.*

Lady Mary Worthly

99

The rule with pants is this: they must fall
gracefully all the way down from your
waistline to your ankles in a straight line.
If something breaks that fall, the pants don't
fit right.

100

Look for long, simple dresses with buttons
down the front.

101

In choosing blouses and dresses, select a
vertical V neckline, rather than a round or
square neckline. The V neckline helps
lengthen and slim the figure.

102

If your neck, shoulders and arms are slender, treat yourself to a one-shouldered evening gown. The eye is encouraged upwards — which is helpful.

103

A man's shirt worn over a swimsuit looks great and can cover up problem areas when relaxing at the pool. Roll up the sleeves and have some fun!

Happiness is not having what you want. It's wanting what you have.

Unknown

104

The duster coat is a must in your wardrobe.
The look is long and lean, but it must drape
well and not overpower. Wear it open.

105

Try to buy natural fabrics that breathe such
as cotton or linen, rather than polyester.
Being comfortable in your clothing,
especially in hot weather, is a must.

106

The tunic dress, with its long, narrow top,
works for all body shapes. Look for a
hemline that doesn't flare.

107

For those who are wide in the hips, wear cap sleeves on a top or dress. They help broaden the shoulder line, which improves your proportions.

108

Knits should never stretch in order to cover the body. Buy it a size or two larger! Then snip off the size tag if that makes you feel better.

One piece of good advice is better than a bag full.

Danish Proverb

109

In general, stick with small, subtle prints only. Bold prints will call attention to a heavy area.

110

For a slimming look, try a swimsuit with attached shorts, or one that looks more like a mini-dress.

111

Your top should always be shorter than your jacket. This gives an uninterrupted line.

112

If you want to wear a belt, the most flattering kind is often the chain belt. It hangs loosely over the hips, it doesn't cinch tightly in at the waist, and it gives a diagonal line.

113

Usually your skirts should not rise above the knee unless your legs look particularly fabulous.

It is an interesting question how far men would retain their relative rank if they were divested of their clothes.

Henry David Thoreau

114

Before purchasing a bra, raise your arms.
Does it ride up and cause a bulge? A good
bra should fall low in the back. Most women
wear bras that are too small, but the right
one can change your entire upper body.

115

Long, semi-wide shorts will make your
legs look slimmer. Also, the hem of your
shorts should not end at the heaviest part of
your legs.

116

Black is slimming, but it can be harsh
for certain skin types. Here is where a
contrasting collar or scarf at the face can
really soften your appearance.

117

A variety of good clothing catalogs are popping up all over. If uncertain, order two sizes of an item to achieve the most flattering fit. These companies are usually gracious about returns.

118

Shorter women will look taller, and therefore slimmer, by avoiding light and dark color combinations. If you don't dress in one color, choose muted shades in the same color range.

He who is ashamed of asking is ashamed of learning.

Danish Proverb

119

By all means resist the blanket-plaid coat, as well as the down coat! They are not figure correcting.

120

If your breast clavicles are prominent, avoid the square-necked blouse.

121

A duffel coat can look great, but keep it on the long side. Also look for the new unlined version.

122

Avoid over-large bracelets. Too much attention at the wrists can widen the look of your hips.

123

Full length sleeves on any garment should fall just below the wrist bone, never longer.

There is an applause superior to that of the multitudes: one's own.

Elizabeth Elton Smith

124

If your ankles are heavy, shoes with wide horizontal straps should be avoided.

125

Particularly with pants, don't be afraid to go a size larger! Pockets and seams should always lie flat.

126

When wearing a business suit, don't let a long skirt drag your look down! Wear the skirt a bit shorter and show some leg. This will also modernize your look.

127

Plump fingers should not be highlighted
with bright fingernail polish or fancy rings.
Oval-shaped nails are best.

128

Pulling your hair back into a severe ponytail
can make your face look plump. Also, let a
little hair fall gently around your face.

*Do not let what you cannot do interfere with what
you can do.*

John Wooden

129

Dresses with color blocking, such as contrasting dark panels running down the sides, are frequently flattering.

130

When buying shoes, look for high quality, natural materials. Fine leather is worth the price. You need good support and comfort. As someone once said: "If your shoes hurt, you wear them on your face."

131

If you are tugging and pulling at clothes —
they don't fit! You shouldn't even be aware
that an article of clothing is on your body.

132

For an uninterrupted line, wear panties that
come to your waistline — like your
pantyhose.

Imagination is more important than knowledge.

Albert Einstein

133

Warm colors — such as red, orange and yellow — tend to make people look larger. Cool colors — such as blue, green and purple — often are slimming. Get your colors analyzed to determine your most complimentary shades.

134

Women with large, broad shoulders should wear a dropped-shoulder style whenever possible to minimize the problem.

135

In general, look for matte textures in clothing. Shiny textures such as satin and metallic will enlarge your silhouette.

136

Find a swimsuit that covers as much skin as possible. Look for a long legline. Beware of the two-piece bikini.

Clothes and courage have so much to do with each other.

Sara Jeanette Duncan

137

The wrap dress or skirt is an excellent choice. Its long, asymmetrical side closure is very flattering — as is the curve at the hemline.

138

If you are bottom heavy, try pants with very subtle front pleats that start several inches below the waistband. Make sure the pleats lie flat.

139

For a trim look on a jacket, seek out flap or slash pockets. Big, square pockets never look as slimming as subtle ones.

140

If you have a double chin, stay away from high collars.

141

Try to find a line of clothing that works great for your figure type. Then generally stick with that designer or designers.

If you think you can, you can. And if you think you can't, you're right.

Mary Kay Ash

142

What you carry is part of your outfit!
Analyze not only your handbag, but your
shoulder bag, briefcase and carry-all so size
does not overwhelm.

143

If wearing a belt, keep it simple in design!
Avoid a large, shiny or decorative buckle.

144

Drawstring pants should look somewhat loose and roomy. They are best in lighter-weight fabrics.

145

It has been said that the eyebrows are the pillars of the face. Well trimmed eyebrows will actually make your face look more lean. But don't go too thin!

Always bear in mind that your own resolution to succeed is more important than any other one thing.

Abraham Lincoln

146

Heavy arms look more attractive in raglan or full sleeves. But avoid cuffs.

147

Bottom-heavy women should look for quality skirts with linings.

148

A long cardigan sweater that falls just below the hips is always flattering — and elegant.

149

The narrower the pant leg, the heavier the fabric can be.

150

If you are broad shouldered, avoid wearing scarves across your shoulders.

In the middle of difficulty lies opportunity.

Albert Einstein

151

A soft-sided briefcase is a better choice for the woman who wants to look a bit slimmer. A hard-sided briefcase will create a bulky, masculine look.

152

Single-breasted blazers are a wardrobe classic. But they can look stiff and add pounds. Choose your fabric wisely and take care with the shoulder fit and length.

153

Be careful of short sleeves. They should at least cover the fullest part of your arm. Long sleeves are often best. Cool, light materials are available.

154

Even in a wedding dress — less is more.
Avoid an elaborate design, big puffy sleeves,
busy details and a top-heavy veil.

155

Do not always wear drab colors. You may
look a bit thinner, but you'll feel drab
as well.

Don't find fault. Find a remedy.

Henry Ford

156

If you have a plump tummy, wear dresses with slightly bloused backs and clothes that fit loosely in the tummy area.

157

The A-line skirt must have a very subtle silhouette to work. A wide hemline will shorten and therefore widen a person.

158

The fabric in a pair of trousers should be soft but strong. The right amount of structure and hold can make all the difference in how flattering a pair of pants looks.

159

If the fabric in your bra, panties or swimsuit loses its elasticity — throw the item out. Think support!

160

To minimize a wide neck, wear a neckline that fits close to the base of your neck.

The difference between good and great is just a little extra effort.

Duffy Daugherty

161

If you look great in hats, wear them! Hats draw the eye up and away from figure flaws. But be careful of large brims if you are short.

162

Any details on the shoulders, such as epaulets, will broaden the silhouette. The military look is best suited for the bottom-heavy woman.

163

Controltop pantyhose now come with stomach-slimming panels that really work. Look for them.

164

In general, buy your blazers, jackets and skirts in neutral colors. But buy your blouses and scarves in bright, intense shades.

165

A lightweight wool gabardine fabric will skim the body beautifully without clinging. Look for it!

The road to success is always under construction.
                                                    Anonymous

166

Pants with a completely flat front are usually best hidden under a long, semi-fitted top.

167

Believe it or not, clothing that softly echoes your shape flatters it!

168

The sailor blouse, with its unique collar and V-neck, is a great way to direct attention upward to your face.

169

Don't carry more than one bag! Try to fit everything into one trim, neat looking bag if possible.

170

Don't wear a swimsuit that is too small. This is a common error. We all know swimsuits are especially unforgiving. So go up a full size. That way your skin won't bulge and the back won't creep up.

When the right thing happens, the whole body knows.

Robert Bly

171

A narrow belt, the same color as your clothes, if worn loosely, will sometimes make the waistline look smaller. But be careful.

172

The sweater dress poses a real risk! It often clings in all the wrong places. Remember, gently flowing, structured clothes are the best way to go.

173

Strangely enough, prints, if very small, can be helpful in a swimsuit. They keep the eye from lingering on trouble spots for too long.

174

All body slimming undergarments should define a woman's curves without constricting them. Body slimmers should breathe, they should stay in place, and they should remain comfortable all day.

175

A thin, body-hugging fabric will always emphasize lumps and bumps. Study fabrics! You'll learn very quickly what is most flattering.

Simplicity is an exact medium between too little and too much.

Sir Joshua Reynolds

176

A brightly colored purse or leather bag can be fun and take attention away from a heavy figure.

177

Square-shaped women should avoid overly masculine, boxy clothes. Please don't fall into that trap!

178

Typically, pleated skirts should be on the long side! But be wary of pleats in general.

179

For comfort, the long, equestrian-style blazer in the new stretch wool is unbeatable. The more stretch anywhere the better! But the garment should have structure.

180

If you have a sweater or a pair of pants that droop after several hours — donate it to the needy at once! Nothing looks worse than a baggy fabric.

How we feel about ourselves is more important than how others feel about us.
                                        Michel Montaigne

181

The wider the skirt, the longer it should be!

182

For the woman with a large bust, avoid a low yoke or smocking in that area.

183

Resist the choker necklace because of its horizontal line.

184

Side vents on a skirt or jacket help fabrics move gracefully for a taller, thinner look.

185

Halter tops require firm arms.

Any garment that makes you feel bad will make you look bad.

Victoria Billings

186

If your ear lobes are large, avoid tiny
earrings.

187

A filmy, sheer shawl can gracefully hide a
top-heavy figure.

188

It may be a search, but choose only a jacket
that fits your figure well. In other words,
don't buy one too large.

189

It is usually best to buy a coat in a solid color for two reasons. First, the one color will be less busy and more slimming. Second, a patterned coat is not as versatile.

190

In warm weather, capris pants can be a smart choice. They are a compromise between shorts and slacks.

No one can make you feel inferior without your consent.

Eleanor Roosevelt

191

If your feet and legs are large, avoid shiny
patent leather shoes.

192

To hide a plump tummy, look for a swimsuit
that is dark on the bottom and light on top.
This will draw the eye upwards.

193

For a vertical line, wear your jacket open,
revealing your blouse underneath.

194

If you have plump knees, choose shorts that
are slightly flared at the bottom.

195

A lining in a jacket helps give it shape and a
more flattering line.

From small beginnings come great things.

Dutch Proverb

196

Your first priority should be to know yourself and your proportions!

197

Dramatic, Hollywood-type sunglasses can be very flattering and will coax the viewer's eye upward. Consider wearing them in your hair as a headband.

198

Does one of your outfits always make you feel slimmer? There is a good reason for it! Analyze why and buy more of the same. People tend to wear only 20% of their wardrobes.

199

Low cut, low rise pants are not recommended. They provide no support and are not very forgiving.

200

Please stay away from very full, pleated skirts. Large pleats add bulk and inches.

The more one judges, the less one loves.

Balzac

201

To distract the eye away from problem hips, try wearing a lightweight sweater over your shoulders. Tie it loosely in front.

202

Carefully placed darts can help beautify and slim the bustline. Make sure they don't pucker.

203

Always cover the elasticized waist with a shirt or blouse top.

204

Wearing leather takes careful planning.
Leather and suede must be soft and the
garment must be well fitted.

205

To de-emphasize a large bust, choose shirts
and sweaters that are soft and loose.

Originality is nothing but judicious imitation.

Voltaire

206

Ornamentation and a colorful design enlarge an area. In other words, if you are large on the top or the bottom, do not call attention to it.

207

For those with large tummies — do not tuck in your blouses or sweaters! Why add a horizontal line where you want it least?

208

One size fits all? Don't believe it! Fit is everything. Try it on.

209

If you find a skirt you love, but it has bulky pockets, consider stitching them down.

210

Important: a blouse or jacket should always button easily, even when you are stretching, bending, sitting or dancing. Buttons in front should never strain to remain buttoned.

Happiness is not a state to arrive at, but a manner of traveling.

Margaret Lee Runbeck

211

Avoid even slightly wrinkled clothes.
Crisply pressed clothes are flattering to
the figure.

212

Accessorize! A long scarf or necklace can
transform an entire outfit instantly and
magically provide a vertical line. Or try
wearing several necklace strands that fall low.

213

Short women should avoid cuffed pants.
They cut height and therefore add pounds.

214

In cooler weather, walking shorts with matching tights look great on most women.

215

Avoid the double-breasted style in a heavy winter coat.

I'm five-feet-four but I always feel six-feet-one, tall and strong.

Yvette Mimieux

216

If your face is round, wear rectangular, navigator or square-shaped frames on your eyeglasses. If your face is square, wear round or oval-shaped frames.

217

Pants and skirts should never, ever fit tightly across a large derriere. Buy the next size up for a loose look.

218

Pay attention to your undergarments! Pretty, feminine underwear will do wonders for your morale.

219

Look for a narrow waistband in a skirt — or a skirt that has no waistband at all.

220

Keep in mind that detailing on clothing, particularly if it is horizontal, will stop the eye from moving upward.

Styles, like everything else, change. Style doesn't.
Linda Ellerbee

221

Empire-waist dresses promote the look of
height. This, in turn, will make you look
thinner. However, large-busted women
should avoid this style.

222

If your hips are wide, dresses and skirts can
be your best friend. You'll also feel more
feminine. Avoid belts with them if possible.

223

Be careful with the size and height of
shoulder pads. They can help balance the
body, but they shouldn't be too high or
too wide.

224

A short, puffed, or decorated sleeve will emphasize a heavy bustline.

225

If you wear a two-piece dress with an overblouse, don't let the overblouse be too billowy.

Self-trust is the first secret of success.

Ralph Waldo Emerson

226

If you like the casual look, stretch jeans are a good option if they're not too tight. And they are really comfortable!

227

Never buy a bra without trying it under a blouse or a sweater first. Get help from a salesperson who really knows the store's product lines.

228

In general, the longer the skirt, the higher the heel! This also works in reverse.

229

Earrings are a great way to distract the eye away from a large bustline.

230

The most complimentary sleeve is usually the simple, set-in sleeve with a shoulder pad.

You must do the thing you think you cannot do.

Eleanor Roosevelt

231

A swing coat looks great over narrow pants. But if it doesn't swing well, don't buy it.

232

In general, keep in mind that a row of wide pleats makes the eye travel horizontally — not a good idea! Although pleats are vertical lines, they don't operate that way.

233

Necklines and shoulder seams should never be over-large or droopy. Shoulder seams should sit on the shoulder bone.

234

You will definitely need a straight black skirt in your wardrobe! It goes with almost everything and black is slimming.

235

A sweater set can look chic on the larger woman — and they come in many great fabrics, such as a buttery cashmere or a cozy cotton.

There is always another time, another second, another hour to do it right.

Andrei Ridgeway

236

Generally stay with the one-piece, one-color swimsuit. You will look more elegant as well.

237

Many women wear shorts that are too small. Beware!

238

Always remember, balance the shoulder line to the hip line.

239

The sweater coat can look great on any woman because of its long, vertical lines. But it should be large enough!

240

Wearing a drop-waist or A-line style dress can minimize a large bust.

With charm, you've got to get up close to see it; style slaps you in the face.

John Cooper Clarke

241

Because unwanted pounds are a special
problem at the pool, choose spandex or
Lycra swimsuits that control the body well.
Look for a heavy fabric that provides girdle-
like support.

242

Women who are a bit heavy in the middle
can look great in jumpsuits — if loosely
belted.

243

Animal prints continue to be popular in the
fashion world, but they emphasize pounds.

244

Try to wear a shoe with at least a medium heel! Save flat shoes for the mall or the beach.

245

If your skirt pinches even a little bit at the waist or hips — beware! Try the next size.

Intelligence consists in recognizing opportunity.

Chinese Proverb

246

A camisole will help give you a smoother, slimmer line when worn under a slightly sheer top.

247

To distract the eye away from a large bustline, wear a high neckline. We all know what a low neckline does after all!

248

If you are tall and want to wear a large, square scarf, place it off center and tie it on the side.

249

For the most part, avoid sleeves that are wide, unless disguising heavy arms. Wide sleeves will call attention to the waist and upper body.

250

A jacket should look great open or closed! Don't plan on wearing it open simply because it fits a bit small.

The shortest answer is doing.

Lord Herbert

251

Do not wear tops and sweaters that bind at the bottom!

252

The cowl neck sweater can really frame a pretty face if the cowl isn't too large. But women with a large bust should avoid them.

253

In general, never hem a dress or skirt mid-calf. Doing so will only emphasize the widest part of your calves.

254

Keep the crease in your pants nice and crisp!
A crease provides a great vertical line. Good
fabric will make it easier to maintain.

255

If you have a large neck or chin, avoid
wearing a bulky turtleneck.

*There is no duty we so much underrate as the
duty of being happy.*

Robert Louis Stevenson

256

The stronger your coloring, the more vibrant
the accent color you can wear. Again, a
bright color will distract from figure flaws.

257

Full-busted women may want to consider
the "Minimizer Bra." It is designed for
ultimate, maximum support.

258

Long, crew neck sweaters look great worn
over slim pants or leggings!

259

The fitted, or hacking jacket, is not for the woman with large hips.

260

Look for structure in a coat. Completely unstructured outer garments will make you look shapeless.

Boldly ventured is half won.

German Proverb

261

Quite tall, somewhat larger women should wear a solid top with a subtly patterned bottom, or vice versa.

262

Wearing scooped neck tops can minimize wide shoulders.

263

A great haircut can do wonders for a plump face! Go to a styling expert and take the time to transform yourself. Also consider putting some light highlights in your hair.

264

To minimize a large bust, look for a dress
that buttons in the back rather than in front.

265

When it fits right, the straight skirt — with
its slim lines — can look terrific on you!
Wear it often.

*The French call it trompe l'oeil — in other words,
to fool the eye.*

French Term

266

Buttons on a jacket can either be a plus or a minus. They should provide a clean, uncluttered, vertical line and be of good quality. Avoid large, shiny buttons.

267

To make a foot look more narrow and slim, select a tapered toe instead of a rounded one. But don't cramp the foot of course.

268

Have some fun with hair ornaments such as combs, barrettes and bands! They will distract the eye away from problem areas.

269

Shop in men's stores for classic, roomy shirts and sweaters! Just make sure they fit correctly in the shoulders and sleeves.

270

If the buttons, zippers, pockets and other design elements on your outfit are small — you will also look smaller. The exception is that a large woman should not wear a tiny pin.

Borrowed clothes are either too tight or too loose.

Philippine Proverb

271

The eye always stops at a skirt hemline because it adds a dreaded horizontal line. Therefore, try to keep skirts as narrow as possible at the hem.

272

For some odd reason, diagonal lines near the bust are frequently flattering.

273

Buy pants to fit your hips! The waistline can be easily taken in.

274

If you are wearing a scarf, avoid the further distraction of large earrings.

275

Stretch pants with a cotton/Lycra blend will provide more support and coverage than thin leggings that cling too much.

Be happy. It's one way of being wise.

Colette

276

If your neck is wide, avoid a straight, blunt
haircut in the back.

277

The shirt jacket can be a real find! It has
vertical lines, cutaway sides for wide hips, and
it goes with almost all skirts and pants.

278

Double-breasted blazers are fine for the tall
woman — but only if the fabric is graceful
and soft. Avoid them in tweed and other
heavy materials.

279

A one-color pantsuit, with a simple blouse, can be slimming on anyone — if the fit is right.

280

To help hide bulges, try to choose pants with a lining.

To profit from good advice requires more wisdom than to give it.

John Churton Collins

281

A safari jacket can be smashing! Look for a supple fabric that isn't too stiff. Also look for one with some length.

282

Coats with prominent seaming in a horizontal line will actually add extra pounds.

283

Always cover up a large bottom. Jackets, vests and tops will all do the trick.

284

Consider purchasing a sports bra for
everyday wear. It will dramatically reduce
your upper silhouette.

285

If your legs are heavy, avoid busy, patterned
stockings.

*The old woman I shall become will be quite
different from the woman I am now. Another I is
beginning.*

Georges Sand

286

Vertical lines can be added in a number of subtle ways: in the trim, in the seams, and in the tiniest of details. Consider adding something yourself!

287

To distract the eye, repeat your accent color in your outfit, such as in your earrings or scarf.

288

Find yourself a flattering negligee to wear around the house, even if you live alone. You should feel pretty as often as possible in order to permanently boost your self esteem.

289

A matching tam, with the crown raised a bit high for the shorter woman, can direct attention away from figure flaws. Also add a pretty pin to your tam if you wish.

290

Remember that your clothes are a reflection of your inner being. So wear a comfortable blazer instead of an old sweatshirt. You'll feel better about yourself all day long.

A problem well stated, is a problem half solved.

Charles Kettering

291

To elongate your figure, choose your shoes and bag in the same general color.

292

Long hair shortens the figure. Therefore, short hair can look smart if your weight is a bit of a problem. But avoid a severe style. Don't cut it too short!

293

A large, wide belt will make your breasts look even larger.

294

Tartan plaids may be good for school uniforms, but they definitely are not flattering to the figure.

295

When breasts are heavy, sleeves should be designed to fall below the bustline — never at the bustline.

Be yourself. The world worships the original.

Ingrid Bergman

296

If your legs are an asset, a long slit skirt can be sexy and distract the eye away from trouble spots.

297

Blouson tops need shoulder pads and should be made with a graceful fabric. The low waistband should fall in a relaxed manner all around.

298

Buy clothes that flatter your figure right now! Don't plan on losing weight to look good in that new outfit. You can always have it taken in later.

299

Flat, side-slash pockets will distract the eye away from a large tummy.

300

Vertical stripes — almost always a good idea — need not be bold. Even subtle vertical pin stripes will make a person look thinner.

If all the flowers wanted to be roses, nature would lose her springtime beauty, and the fields would no longer be decked out with little wildflowers.

Thèrése of Lisièux

301

Avoid fussy hair, fussy clothes, fussy jewelry — fussy everything! Busyness adds pounds.

302

Short, round-shaped women will look taller and thinner by dressing all in one color. In fact, so will all women!

303

Do not wear earrings that dangle. They will shorten and widen the neck.

304

The slightly flared skirt looks well on the bottom-heavy woman — if it is long and supple.

305

Quality, bias–cut dresses can take off as much as ten pounds.

Fashion changes, style evolves.

Hara Estroff Marano

306

Camisoles — found in the lingerie section —
often come with sewed in shoulder pads to
help balance your silhouette.

307

Did you know those big companies like
Lee and Levi make jeans for all figure types?
Go shopping more often and see what is
out there!

308

Generally, think in terms of a long, lean,
unbroken silhouette.

309

Very slightly pleated pants can help minimize wide hips.

310

Long, multiple strands of pearls, graduated in size, provide an elegant illusion to help the neck look longer and slimmer.

The fragrance always remains in the hand that gives the rose.

Heda Bejar

311

Clothes should fit at all critical points: in the neck, shoulders, sleeves and leg bottoms!

312

The mandarin coat, with its stand-up collar, has great vertical lines and adds height.

313

Cuffs on pants will add two more horizontal lines, but at times you may want them. Just keep them as small as possible.

314

It may be fashionable to partially bare breasts and tummies for a casual look. However, this trend can be very unflattering.

315

Slightly exaggerated shoulder pads will make your waist — and hips — look more trim.

Friendship with oneself is all important, because without it one cannot be friends with anyone else in the world.

Eleanor Roosevelt

316

No matter what — avoid stiff, heavy fabrics. They add bulk. Choose fabrics on the soft side that are flat and drape well.

317

This bears repeating: wear the right foundation garments. A good bra can take five pounds off of your silhouette.

318

The softly pleated skirt can look attractive on taller women. If the fabric drapes well and is not overpowering, this skirt can be slimming because of its many long vertical lines and roomy fit.

319

If upper arms are a bit flabby, avoid sleeveless tops altogether — unless worn underneath something.

320

Split skirts, also called culottes, are usually flattering to all.

Wisdom without use is fire without warmth.

Swedish Proverb

321

Full bangs broaden a face because of the added horizontal line. But very light, wispy bangs can be flattering and youthful.

322

Throw away all of your tent dresses! Tents are for camping.

323

Avoid borders and bands at your hemline!

324

A shiny face will look more plump. Wear foundation that closely matches your skin tone.

325

To show off great legs, wear bright, daring colors, such as a colorful skirt. Remember: distract, distract!

It is never too late to be what you might have been.

George Eliot

326

Sleeves that are tapered in at the wrist are slimming.

327

Following a fashion fad can be risky! Please resist unless the look really hides pounds.

328

Cover up as much as you like! Never be intimidated into wearing a swimsuit or shorts if you don't want to. Slip into something long and light and fluid instead. Find the courage to dress as you wish!

329

This secret seems obvious or silly — but it works! Simply pretend that you are more slim than you are. You will immediately begin to think, feel, look and move differently.

330

Be creative and have a great time with your wardrobe! Take chances! Your enthusiasm and confidence will be contagious.

Have fun! Misery is optional.

Jean Westcott

BOOK INFORMATION

Dress Thin! may be purchased at a Special Bulk Discount for Company Premiums, Store Promotions, Charity Events and so on.

Book Excerpts and Customized Book Editions can be easily arranged.

Please contact Brainstorm Books.

The Authors are available --and even enjoy-- Interviews, Personal Appearances, and Seminars on related subjects.

BOOK AVAILABILITY

Visit:

- www.dressthin.com
- Any Major Internet Bookseller
- Your Local Bookstore

BRAINSTORM BOOKS
P.O. Box 1005
Thousand Oaks, CA 91358-0005